Why can't I have a Cupcake?

Betsy Childs

Illustrated by Dan Olson

Childpress CB Books

To George,
who never complained.
—B.C.

For the Brown boys.
—D.O.

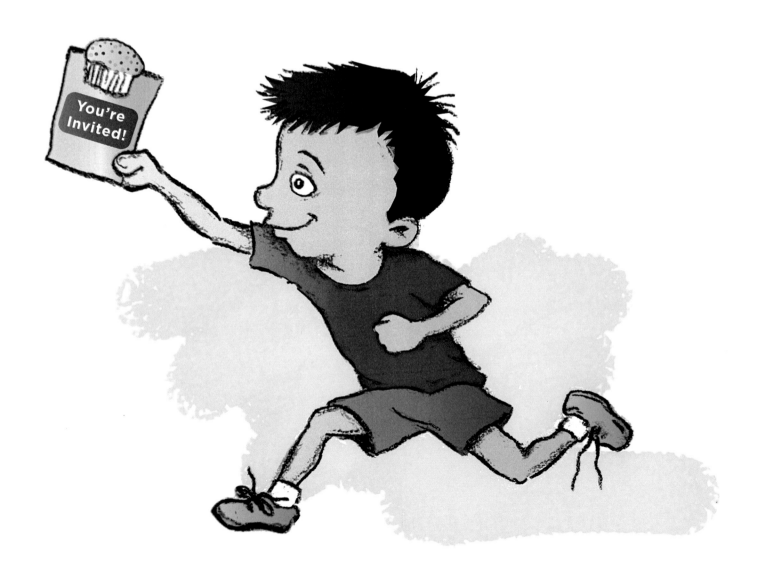

Rory was six years old, and like every six year old, he loved birthday parties.

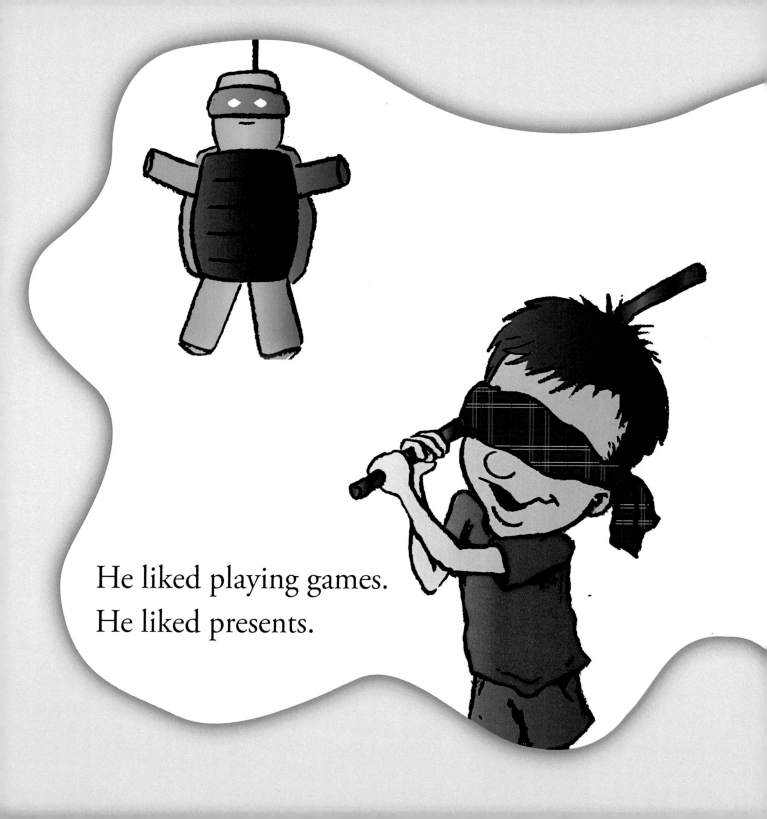

He liked playing games.
He liked presents.

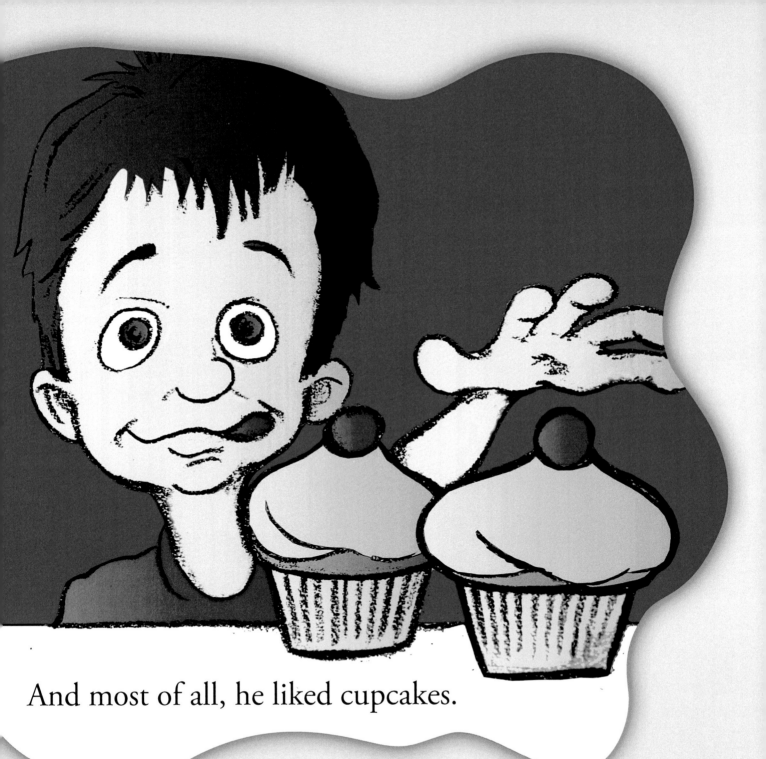

And most of all, he liked cupcakes.

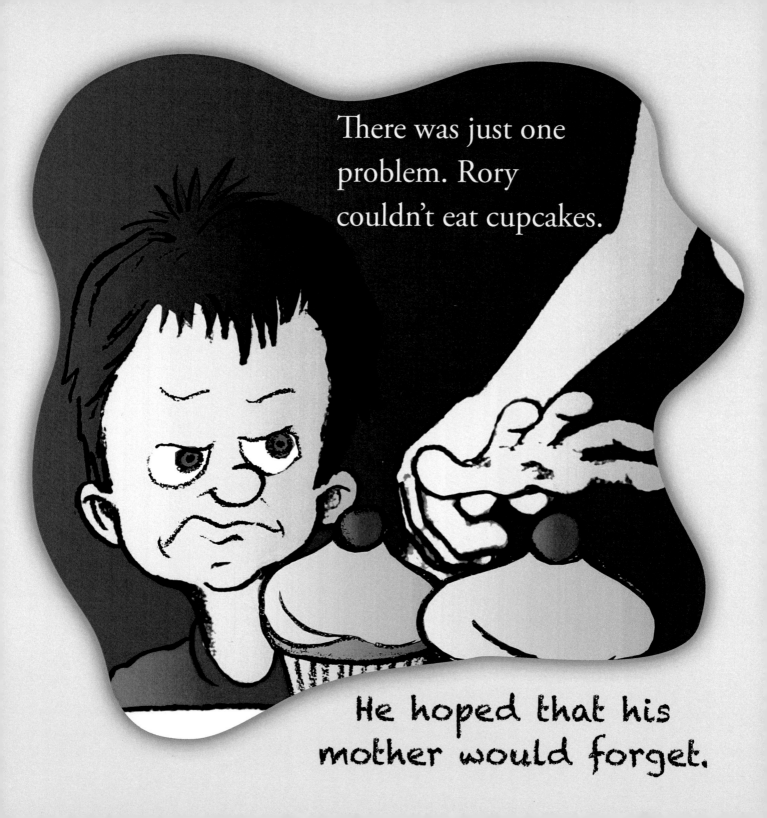

There was just one problem. Rory couldn't eat cupcakes.

He hoped that his mother would forget.

As she helped him get his shoes on to go to Poppy's party, Rory looked out of the corner of his eye and said, **"I am going to eat a chocolate cupcake at the party."** Rory's mother didn't look up as she tied his shoe.

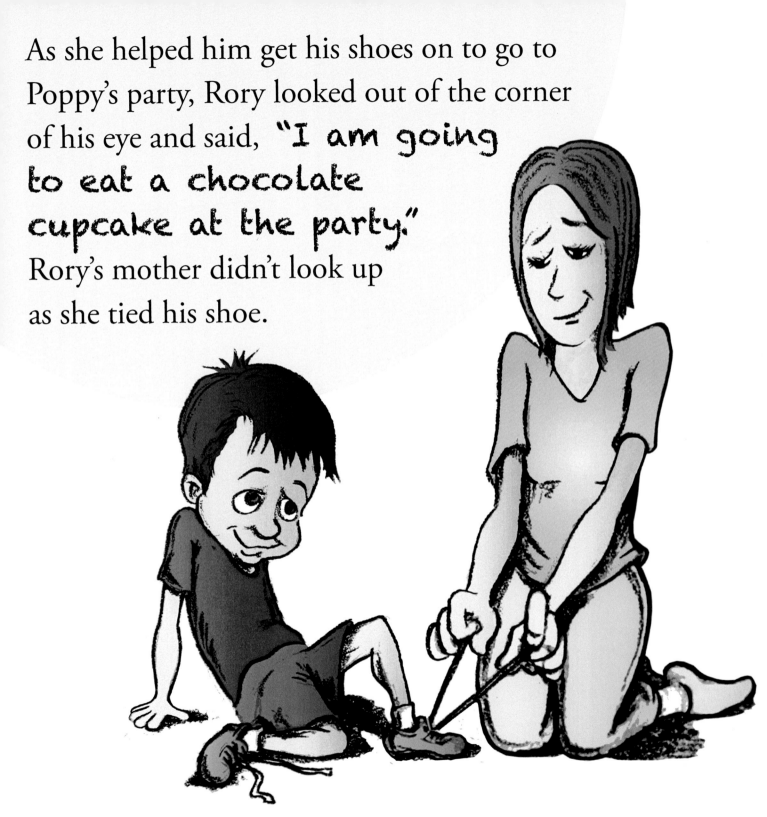

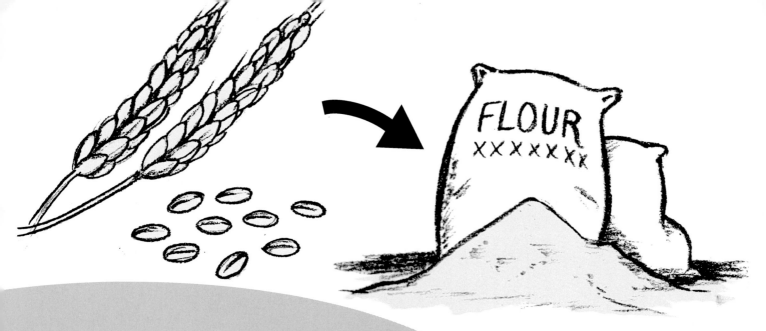

"No, Rory, you can't have a cupcake, remember? Cupcakes are made with flour, and flour has lots of gluten, and when you eat gluten, your tummy hurts."

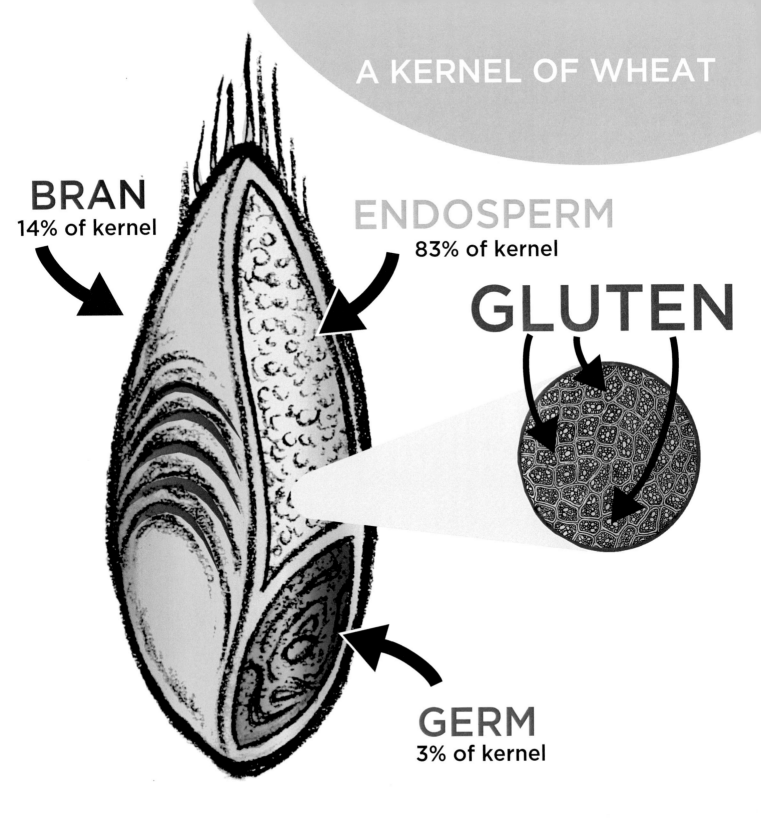

A KERNEL OF WHEAT

BRAN
14% of kernel

ENDOSPERM
83% of kernel

GLUTEN

GERM
3% of kernel

Rory's mother helped him stand up and said, "Do you remember when you ate pancakes last month?

"Pancakes are made of gluten. After you ate them, your tummy hurt all morning, and you had to miss your soccer game because you were ill."

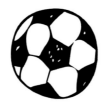

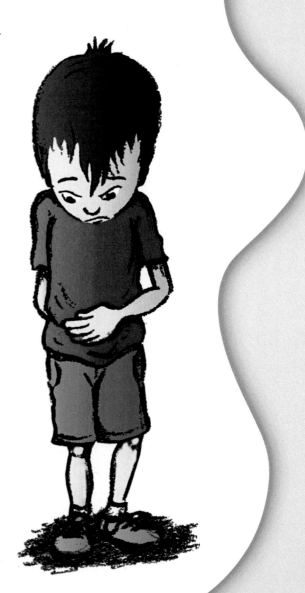

Rory did remember. He remembered what it felt like to have a tummy ache, but he also remembered how much he liked cupcakes. He thought about them all the way to the party.

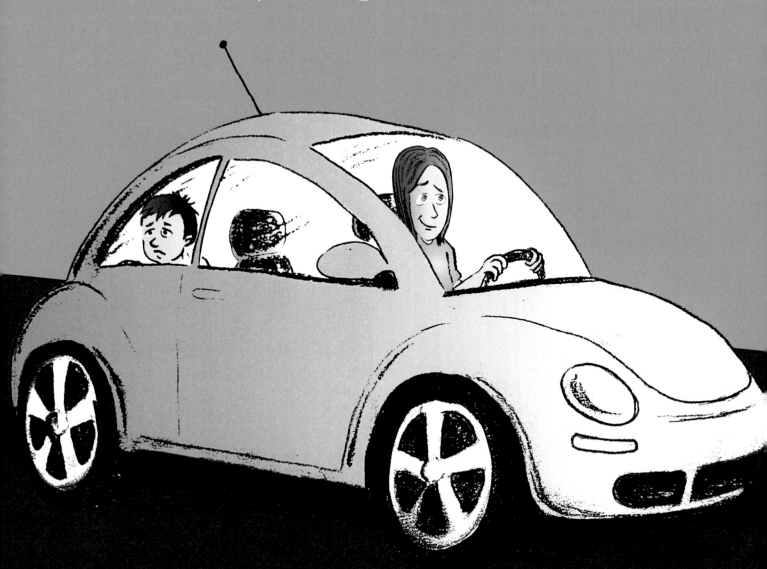

When they arrived at Poppy's house, Rory's mother let him carry the present for Poppy. She also gave him a crispy bar in a baggy.

"You can eat this when they bring out the cupcakes, Rory," she said.

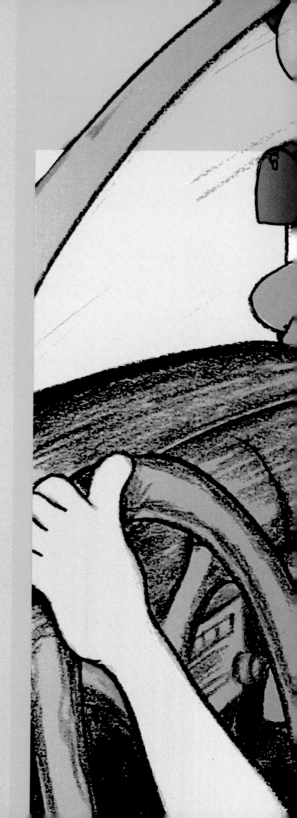

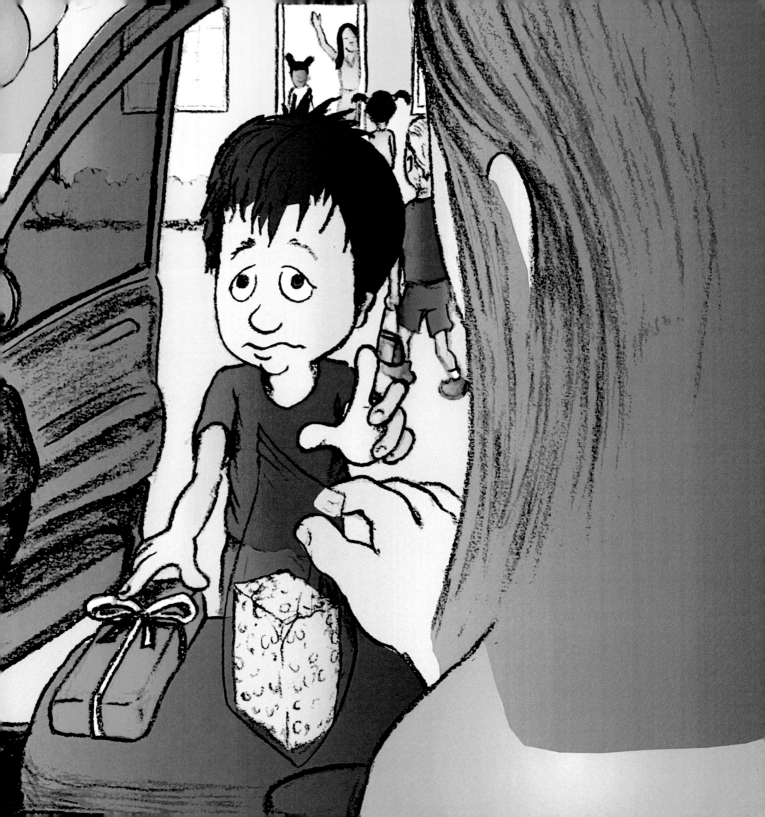

Rory handed Poppy the present and gave the crispy bar to Poppy's mother.

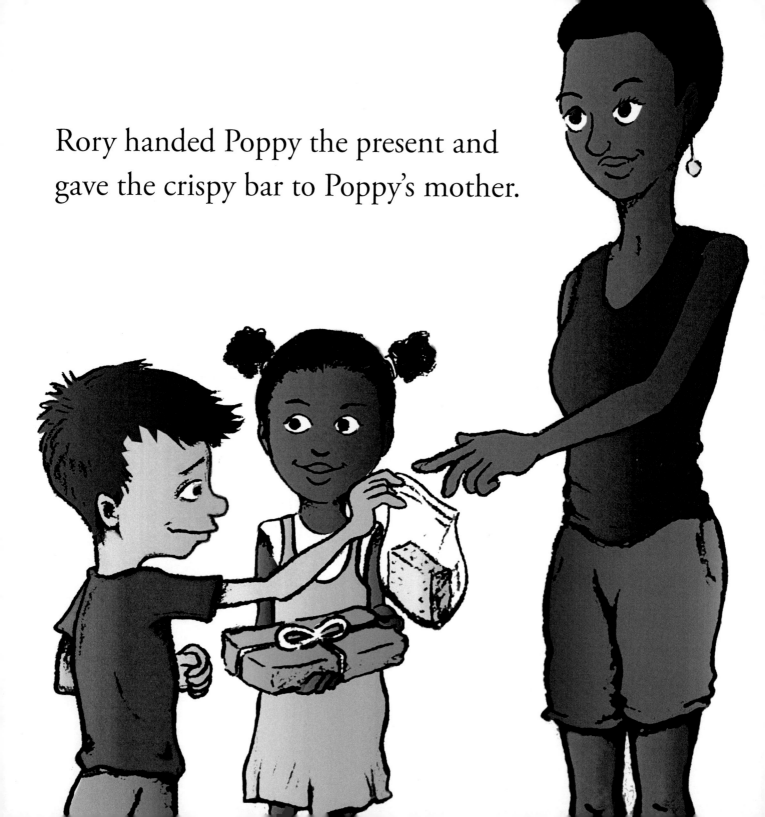

"Thank you, Rory," she said,
"I'll put this with the others."

"Others?" said Rory,
"What others?"

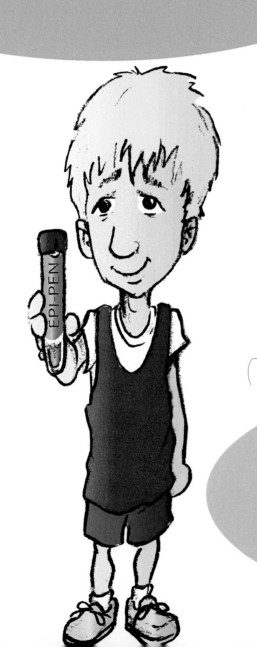

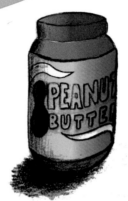

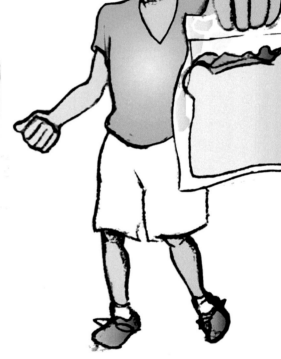

"Well, Celia can't have peanuts, so she brought a tuna sandwich in case we have PB&J."

"Mason brought his epi pen because he is allergic to bee stings."

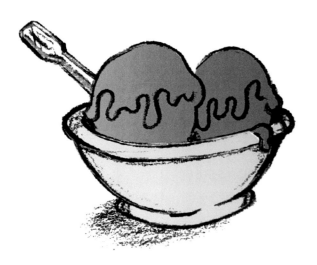

"And Lewis brought a popsicle because he can't have the ice cream. He's allergic to dairy."

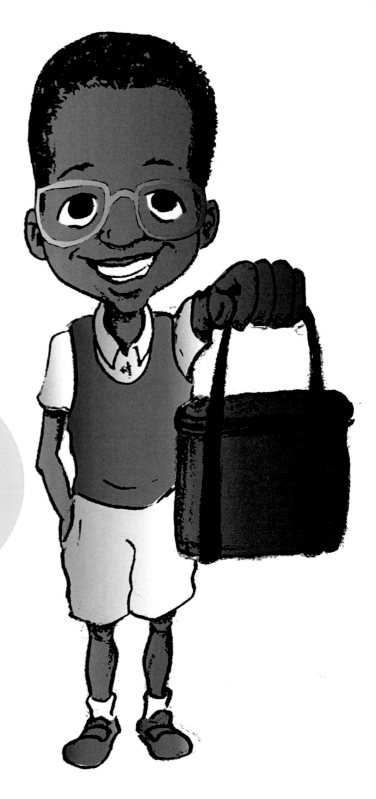

"Lewis
can't have
ice cream?"
Rory said.

He loved ice cream
even more than he
loved cupcakes.

He thought about
that as he stood in
line for pin the nose
on the snowman.

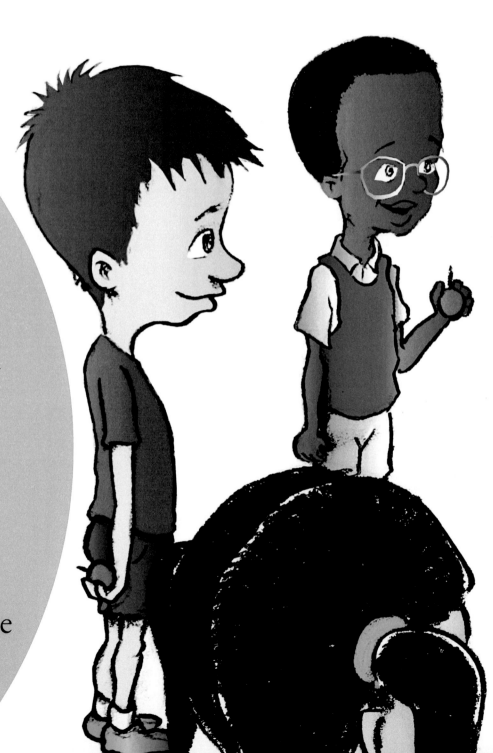

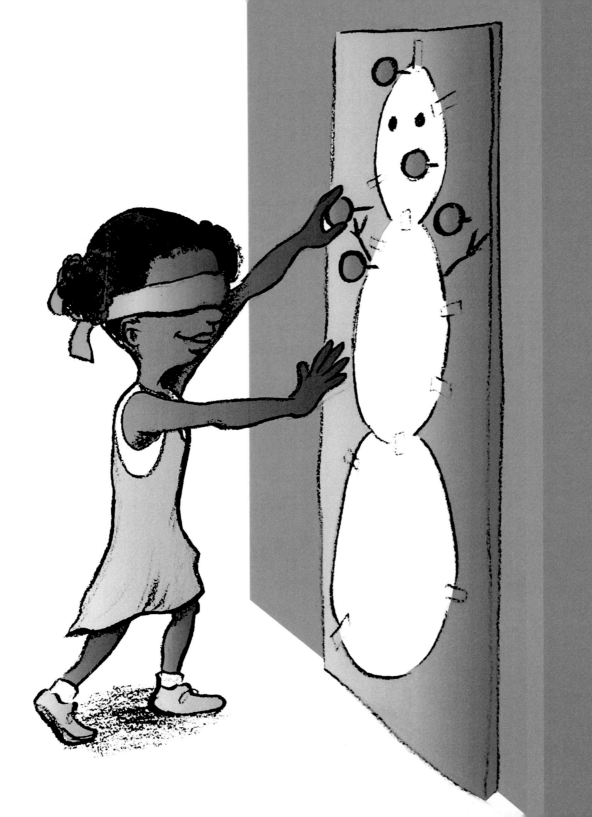

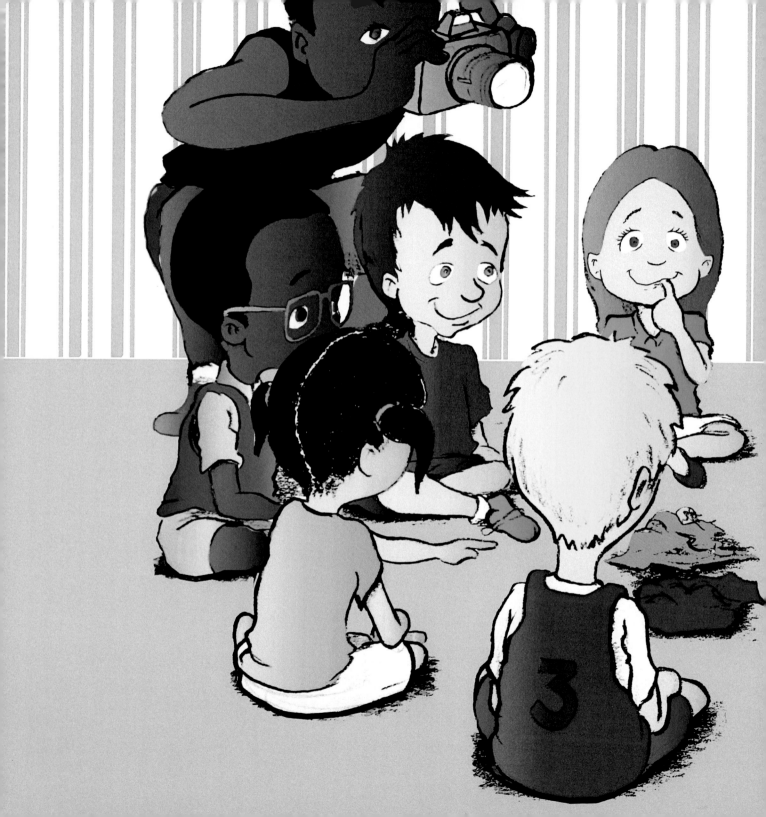

Poppy opened her presents and remembered to say thank you for each one. Rory gave her a new paints set with 44 different colors.

After presents, it was time for ice cream and cake.

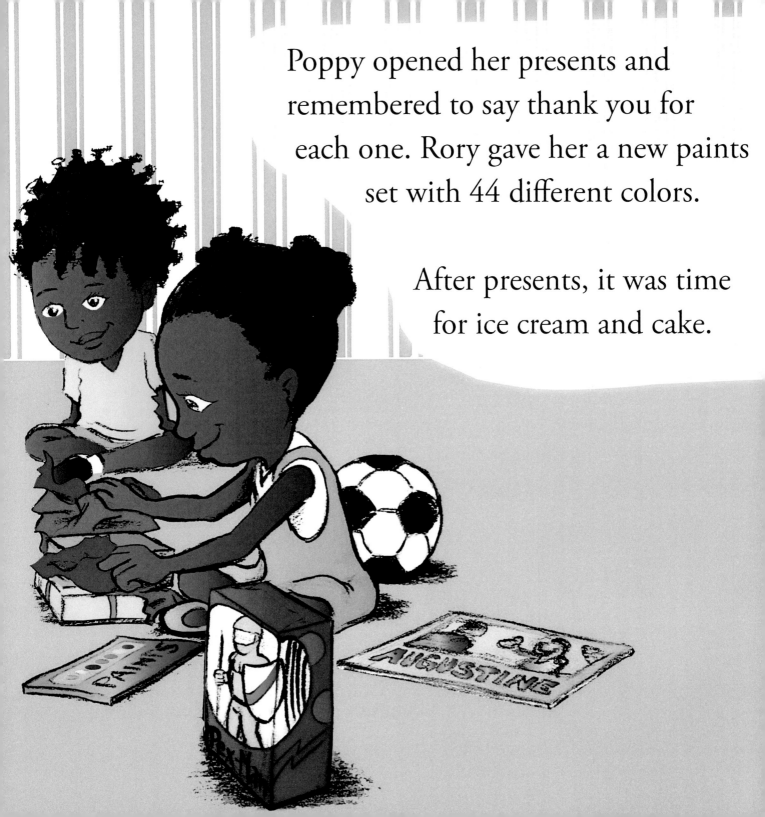

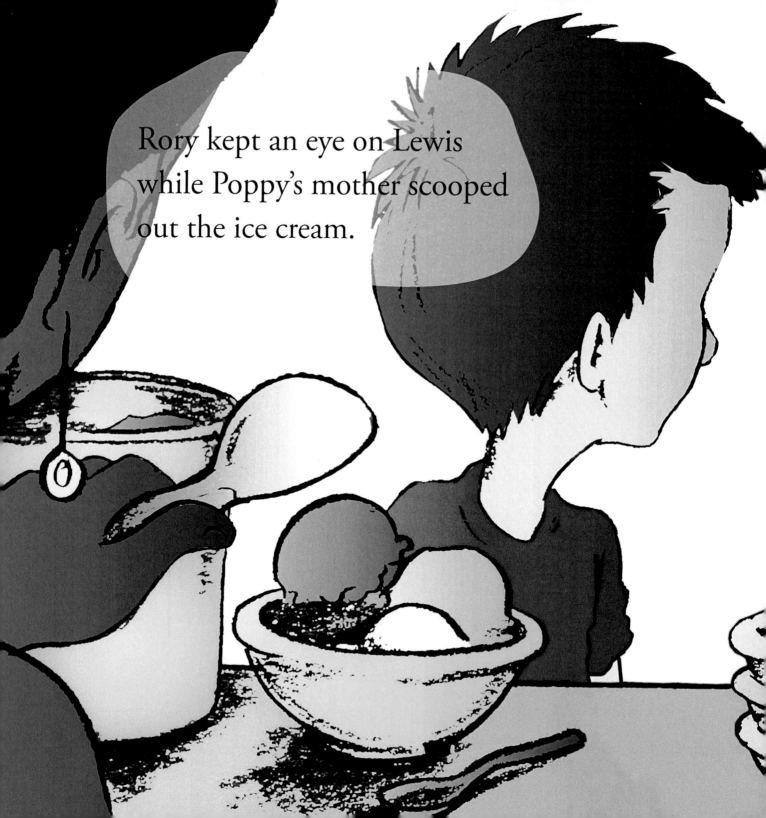

Rory kept an eye on Lewis while Poppy's mother scooped out the ice cream.

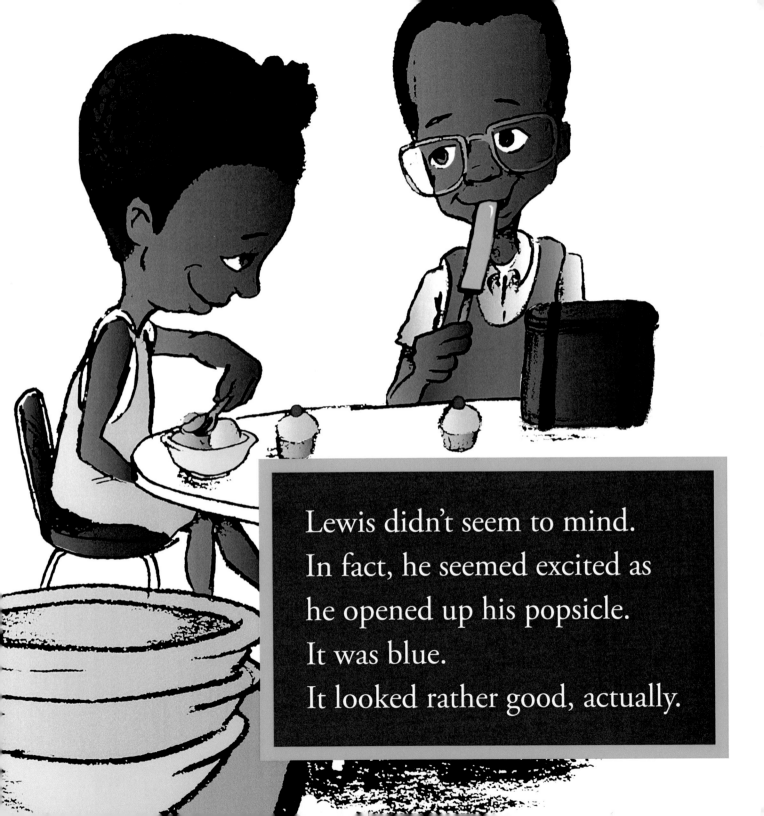

Lewis didn't seem to mind.
In fact, he seemed excited as
he opened up his popsicle.
It was blue.
It looked rather good, actually.

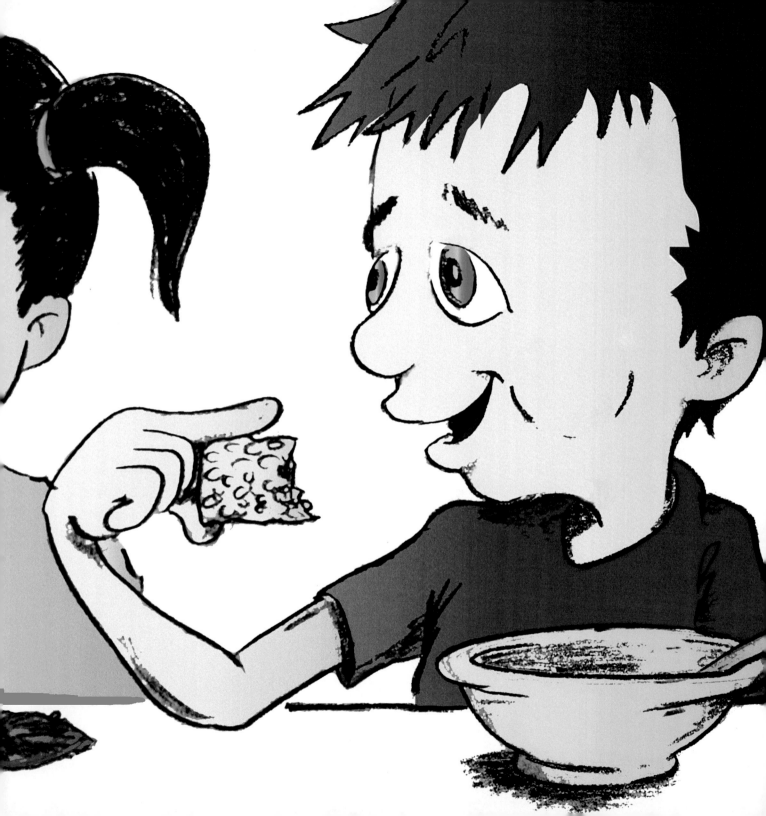

Poppy's mother handed Rory his crispy bar. He ate his ice cream first so that it wouldn't melt.

None of the other children noticed that Rory didn't eat a cupcake.

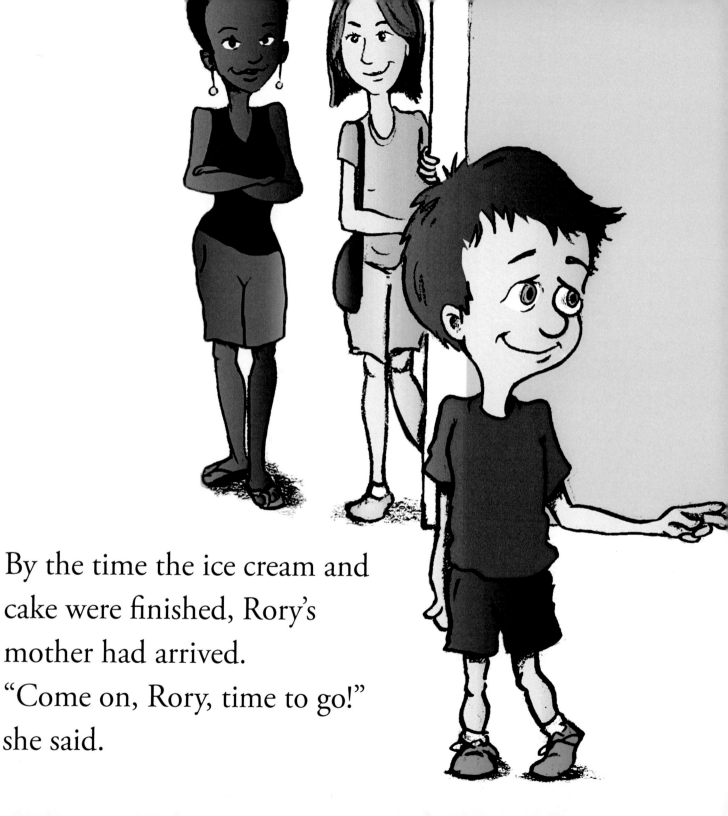

By the time the ice cream and cake were finished, Rory's mother had arrived. "Come on, Rory, time to go!" she said.

Rory found Poppy looking at her new paints set.
"Thank you for inviting me to your party, Poppy," he said.
"You're welcome, Rory," she replied,
"don't forget your favor!"

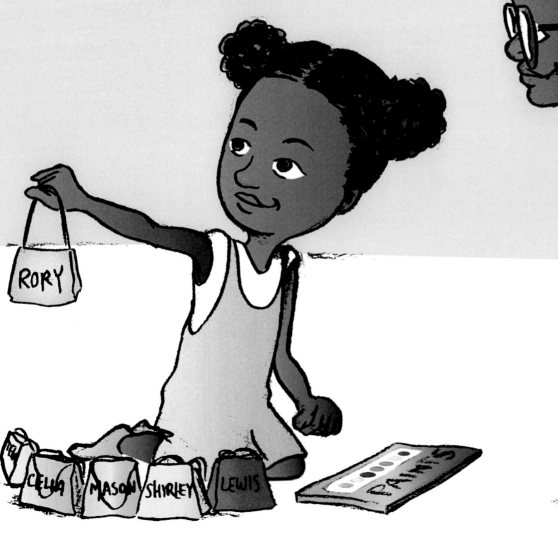
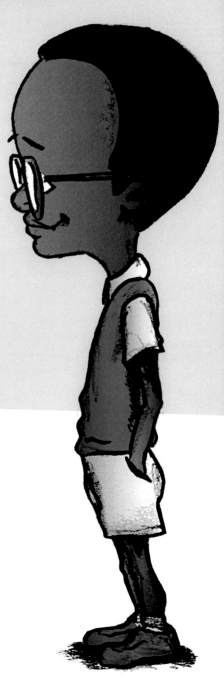

His party favor was a shiny new harmonica. He blew into it as he skipped to the car.

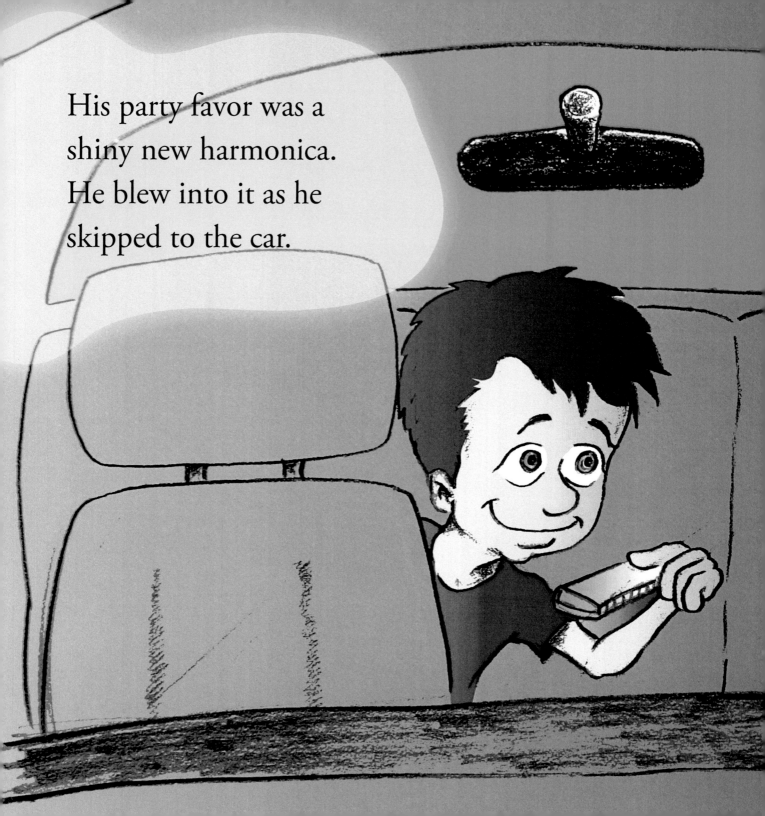

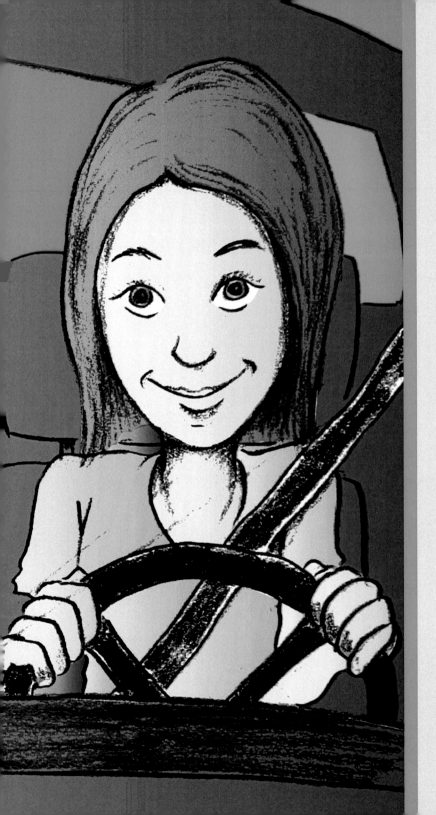

After he buckled up, Rory's mother said, "I have a surprise for you. I found a bakery that makes cupcakes that you can eat.

Would you like to have a cupcake?"

"Are you kidding?" said Rory. "Yippee!"

He would have jumped in the air, but the buckle on his booster kept him in his seat, so instead he just burst out singing:

"Happy birthday to me!"

(which was very silly since it was not his birthday).

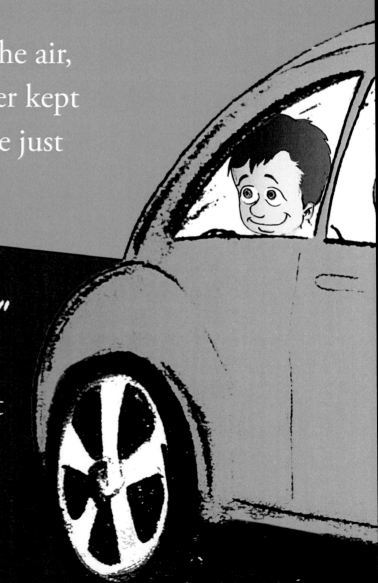

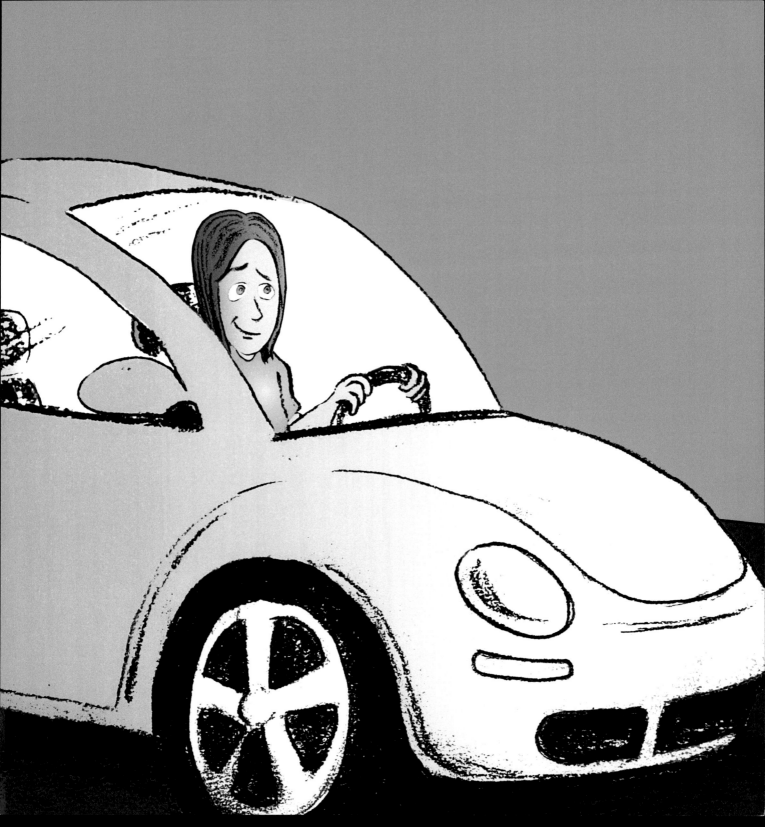

When they went in the bakery a little bell jingled. A nice looking woman came out of the back and stood behind the bakery case. Rory had never seen so many cupcakes in his life.

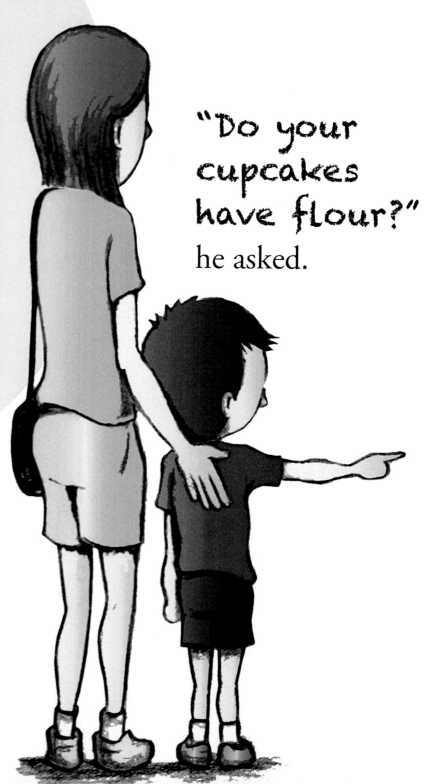

"Do your cupcakes have flour?" he asked.

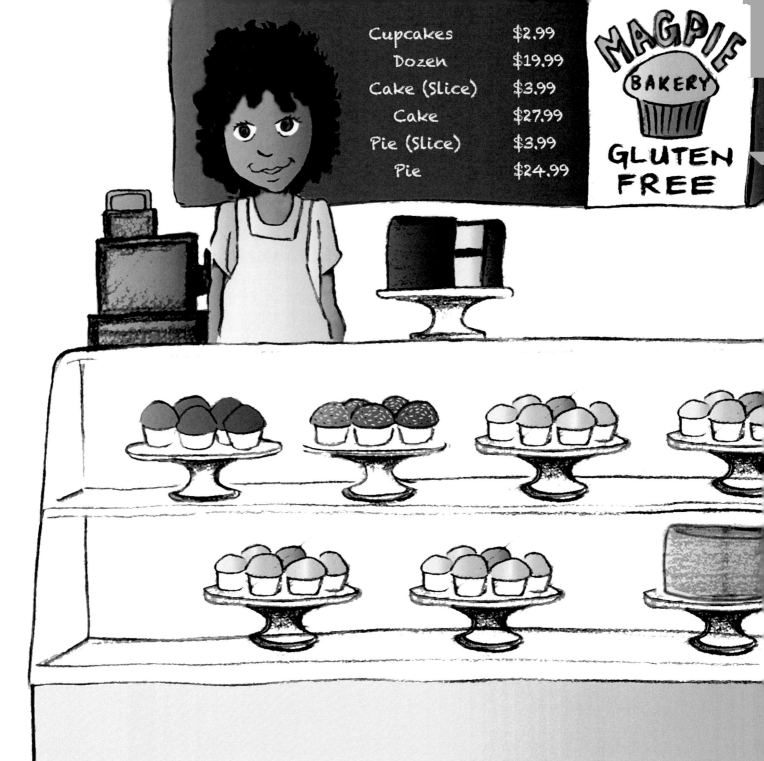

"Yes, they have flour, but I use gluten-free flour. Gluten makes my tummy hurt," said the lady.

"Mine too!" said Rory. "I haven't had a cupcake in forever. I'll take the chocolate one with the sprinkles."

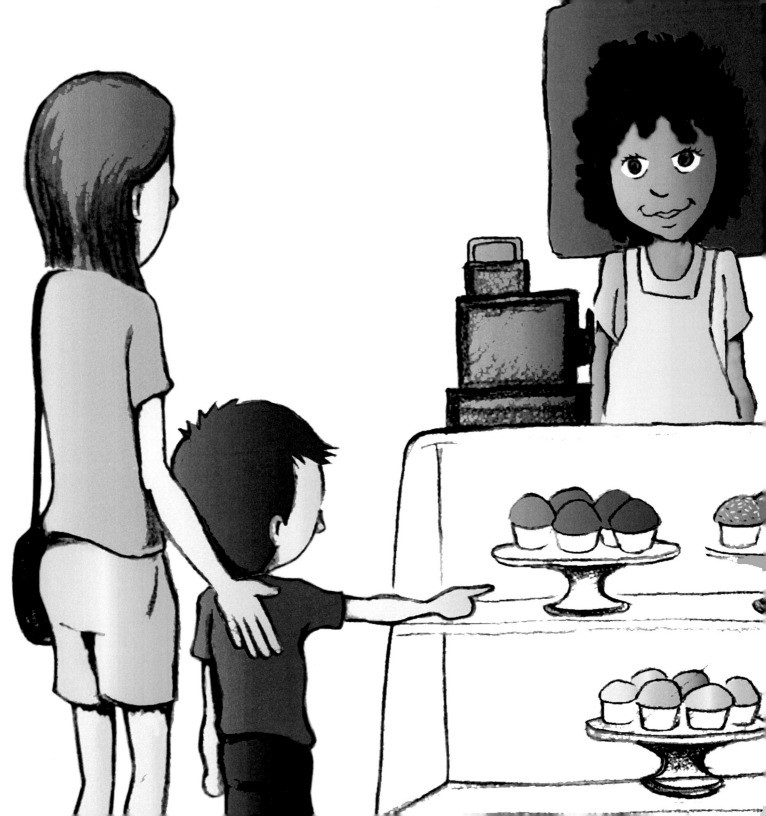

The lady opened the case
and handed Rory the biggest
one. It was so big, he had to
hold it with two hands.

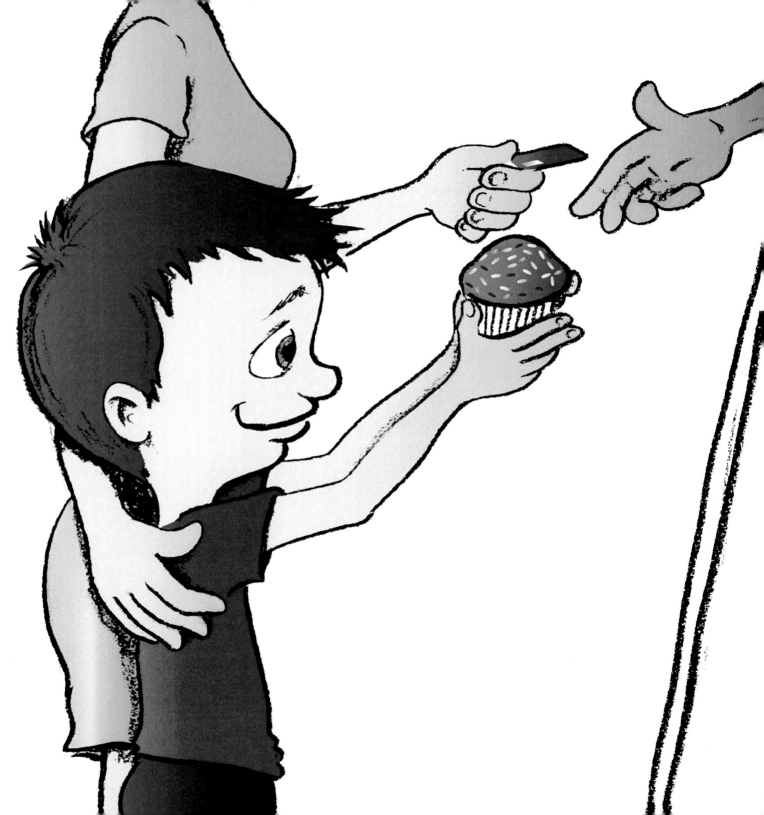

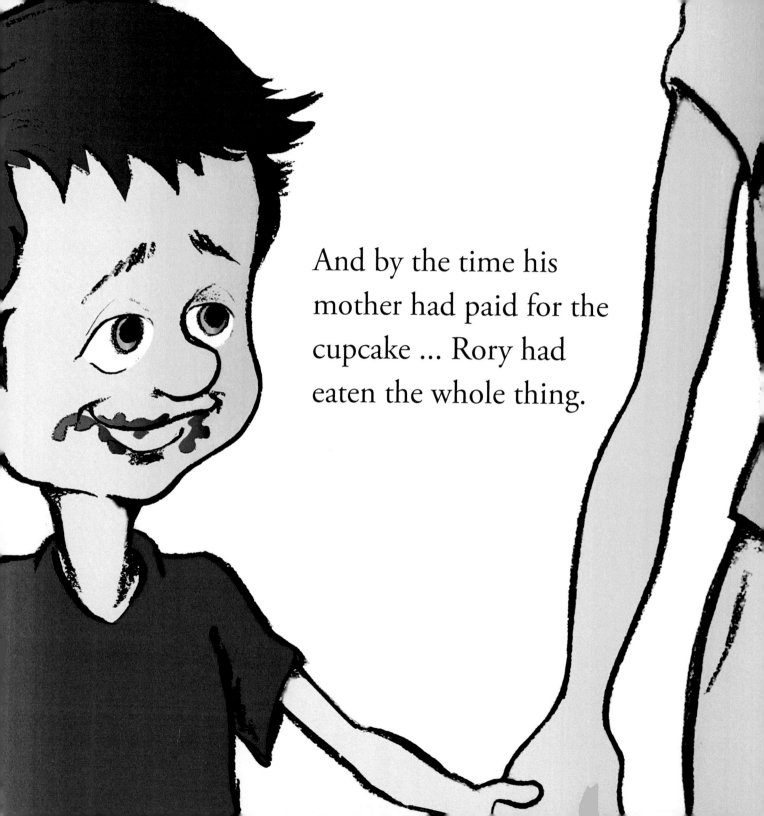

And by the time his mother had paid for the cupcake ... Rory had eaten the whole thing.

The End

Also available from 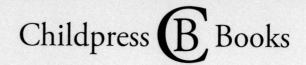Childpress CB Books

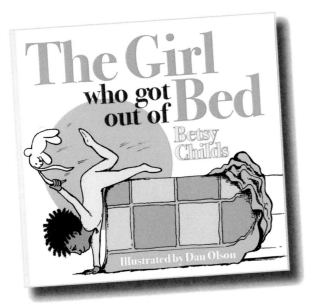

Shirley is a little girl who keeps thinking of reasons to get out of bed. But once she learns the secret to make morning time come, she can't wait for bedtime to roll around again.

Paperback
ISBN-10: 1489595570
ISBN-13: 978-1489595577

Kindle Edition
ASIN: B00DBOYZBM

**$8.99 @ createspace.com/4302316
or @ amazon.com!**

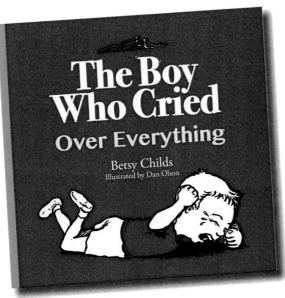

Murray is almost four years old, and he cries over everything. An experience with a slingshot and a sparrow helps him learn that it's okay to cry when you're sad, but it's best not to cry when you're mad. A sweet story and tool to help children learn self-control!

Paperback
ISBN-10: 1467996440
ISBN-13: 978-1467996440

Kindle Edition
ASIN: B006QWS1J8

**$8.99 @ createspace.com/3734469
or @ amazon.com!**

The mission of Childpress Books is to assist parents in forming the moral imagination of children through well-crafted books.

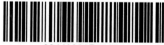

23440926R00024

Made in the USA
San Bernardino, CA
19 August 2015